Weight loss beginners Guide 2024: Discover Simple Steps and Practical Tips for Effectiveness and Start Your Health Transformation Today.

Sharon S. Lent

All rights reserved. No part of the publication maybe reproduced,distributed or transmitted in any form or by any means, including photocopying, recording, or other electronic or mechanical methods, without the prior written permission of the publisher, expect in the case of brief quotation embodied in critical reviews and certain other non-commercial uses permitted by copy right law.

Copyright (Sharon S. Lent),(2023).

Table of Contents

INTRODUCTION

Welcome to the Weight Loss Beginners Guide 2024! Embarking on a journey towards a healthier, more balanced lifestyle is a commendable endeavor. This guide is designed to provide you with essential insights and practical strategies to kickstart your weight loss journey effectively. Whether you're new to the concept of healthy living or seeking fresh perspectives, these pages will guide you through the fundamentals of nutrition, goal setting, meal planning, exercise, and more. Get ready to embrace positive changes and cultivate habits that will contribute to your well-being. Let's begin this transformative adventure together.

Knowledge is a powerful tool on your weight loss journey. Explore recommended resources and further reading to deepen your understanding of nutrition, fitness, and overall well-being. From reputable websites to insightful books, this section provides a curated list of resources to support your ongoing education and growth

Congratulations on reaching the conclusion of the Weight Loss Beginners Guide 2024! Armed with knowledge, strategies, and a newfound sense of empowerment, you are well-equipped to navigate your weight loss journey. Remember that progress is a journey, not a destination. Embrace the positive changes you've implemented and continue to cultivate habits that contribute to your well-being. May your path to a healthier you be fulfilling, rewarding, and filled with sustainable success.

Understanding Weight Loss

Understanding weight loss is a multifaceted exploration that goes beyond the simple concept of shedding pounds. It involves comprehending the intricate interplay of factors influencing our body composition, metabolism, and overall well-being. Let's delve into the fundamental aspects of understanding weight loss.

1. Energy Balance: The Core Principle

At its core, weight loss is governed by the principle of energy balance. This concept revolves around the relationship between the calories consumed through food and beverages and the calories expended through basal metabolic rate (BMR) and physical activity. To lose weight, the calories burned must exceed the calories consumed, creating a calorie deficit.

2. The Role of Macronutrients and Micronutrients

While counting calories is essential, the quality of those calories matters too. Understanding the roles of macronutrients (carbohydrates, proteins, and fats) and micronutrients (vitamins and minerals) is crucial. Each plays a specific role in supporting bodily functions, and a balanced intake is vital for overall health during the weight loss process.

3. Metabolism: Unraveling the Mysteries

Metabolism, often used as a catch-all term, encompasses the processes by which our bodies convert food into energy. Basal metabolic rate (BMR) represents the energy expended at rest. Factors such as age, gender, genetics, and muscle mass influence metabolism. Contrary to common belief, metabolism is not static and can be influenced through lifestyle choices, including diet and exercise.

4. Sustainable vs. Fad Diets: Navigating the Landscape

The weight loss industry is flooded with a myriad of diets, ranging from trendy fads to scientifically-backed approaches. Differentiating between sustainable, evidence-based strategies and quick-fix solutions is crucial. Understanding that a one-size-fits-all approach doesn't exist and that lifestyle changes are more effective in the long run is key to successful weight loss.

5. Body Composition: Beyond the Scale

Weight loss isn't solely about the number on the scale. Body composition, which considers the ratio of fat to lean mass, provides a more nuanced understanding. Building and preserving lean muscle mass is integral to a healthy body composition. Strength training and resistance exercises play a significant role in achieving this balance.

6. Hormones and Hunger: The Internal Regulators
Hormones, the body's messengers, play a vital role in weight regulation. Leptin and ghrelin, for instance, influence hunger and satiety. Understanding how these hormones respond to factors like sleep, stress, and nutritional choices can help in making informed decisions that support weight loss goals.

7. Emotional Eating and Mindful Practices
Acknowledging the emotional aspect of eating is crucial in understanding weight loss. Emotional eating, often triggered by stress, boredom, or other emotions, can impact food choices. Adopting mindful eating practices, such as being present during meals and recognizing true hunger cues, fosters a healthier relationship with food.

8. Slow and Steady Wins the Race: Realistic Expectations
Weight loss is a gradual process, and setting realistic expectations is paramount. Rapid weight loss may lead to muscle loss and nutritional deficiencies. Aiming for a steady, sustainable pace allows the body to adapt positively and increases the likelihood of maintaining the achieved results.

9. Personalized Approaches: The Unique You

Recognizing that individuals respond differently to various approaches is a cornerstone of understanding weight loss. Factors such as genetics, lifestyle, and health conditions influence how bodies react to diet and exercise. Tailoring strategies to suit your unique circumstances ensures a more effective and personalized weight loss journey.

10. Long-term Lifestyle Changes: Beyond the Finish Line

Understanding weight loss isn't just about reaching a specific weight goal; it's about embracing lasting lifestyle changes. Establishing habits that are maintainable, enjoyable, and conducive to overall well-being ensures that the benefits of your efforts extend far beyond the initial weight loss phase.

Understanding weight loss is a dynamic and multifaceted process that goes beyond mere calorie counting. It involves grasping the intricate relationships between nutrition, metabolism, hormones, and emotional well-being. By adopting a holistic approach that considers individual differences and focuses on sustainable lifestyle changes, you pave the way for a healthier, more fulfilling journey towards achieving and maintaining your weight loss goals.

Setting realistic goals

is a crucial foundation for a successful and sustainable weight loss journey. Here's a breakdown of key principles to guide you in establishing achievable objectives:

1. Specificity is Key

Define your goals with precision. Instead of a vague objective like "lose weight," specify the amount you aim to lose and in what timeframe. For example, "Lose 10 pounds in the next eight weeks" provides a clear and measurable target.

2. Make Goals Measurable

Measurable goals enable you to track progress. Instead of a broad goal such as "exercise more," set a measurable target like "Walk 30 minutes every day." This allows for clear assessment and adjustment as needed.

3. Attainability Matters

While ambition is commendable, goals should be realistically attainable. Consider your lifestyle, commitments, and potential obstacles. Setting unattainable goals may lead to frustration and hinder long-term success. Opt for gradual, achievable milestones that align with your capabilities.

4. Relevant and Realistic Timeframes

Establish a timeframe that aligns with your overall objective. Short-term goals should contribute to long-term success. For instance, if your ultimate goal is to lose 20 pounds, set realistic monthly targets that contribute to this overarching aim.

5. Consider Behavioral Changes

Recognize that successful weight loss often requires behavioral changes. Set goals that encompass healthy habits such as mindful eating, regular exercise, and sufficient sleep. Focusing on behavior rather than just outcomes enhances the sustainability of your objectives.

6. Break Down Larger Goals

Divide larger goals into smaller, manageable steps. If your ultimate aim is significant weight loss, breaking it down into smaller increments makes the process less overwhelming. Achieving these smaller goals provides a sense of accomplishment and motivation.

7. Flexibility for Adaptation

Life is dynamic, and circumstances may change. Allow flexibility in your goals to adapt to unexpected challenges or opportunities. Instead of viewing setbacks as failures, consider them opportunities for learning and adjustment.

8. Celebrate Achievements

Celebrate your victories, both big and small. Acknowledging achievements reinforces positive behavior and motivates further progress. This could be treating yourself to a non-food reward or simply reflecting on your accomplishments.

9. Align with Personal Values
Connect your goals with your values. If improving overall health is a primary motivator, set goals that align with this value. This connection enhances commitment and makes the journey more meaningful.

10. Regularly Evaluate and Adjust
Regularly assess your progress and adjust goals as needed. If you consistently surpass objectives, consider setting more challenging ones. Conversely, if progress is slower than anticipated, evaluate potential barriers and make adjustments to your approach.

Setting realistic goals involves specificity, measurability, attainability, relevance, and timeframes. Behavioral changes, flexibility, celebrations, alignment with personal values, and regular evaluations contribute to a well-rounded goal-setting strategy. By adopting these principles, you create a roadmap that not only guides your weight loss journey but enhances the likelihood of sustained success.

CHAPTER 1
Nutrition Basics

Nutrition forms the foundation of a healthy life and is necessary in any weight loss trip. Then are abecedarian nutrition basics to guide you

1. Balanced Diet The Foundation

A balanced diet includes a variety of foods from all food groups. This encompasses ;

** **Fruits and Vegetables** ** Rich in vitamins, minerals, fiber, and antioxidants.

** **Whole Grains** ** Sources of complex carbohydrates, fiber, and essential nutrients.

** **Proteins** ** spare flesh, flesh, fish, sap, nuts, and tofu for muscle health and malnutrition.

** **Dairy or Alternatives** ** Calcium-rich sources for bone health.

** **Healthy Fats** ** Avocado, nuts, seeds, and olive oil painting give essential adipose acids.

2. Portion Control Quality and Quantity Matter

Understanding portion sizes is pivotal. Indeed healthy foods can contribute to weight gain if consumed exorbitantly. Use visual cues, similar as the size of your win or a sundeck of cards, to gauge applicable portions.

3. Hydration Water is Vital

Acceptable hydration is essential for overall health and can prop in weight loss. Aim to drink plenitude of water throughout the day, and consider choosing water as your primary libation.

4. aware Eating Savor Every Bite

Rehearsing aware eating involves being present during refections, paying attention to hunger and wholeness cues, and savoring each bite. This approach fosters a healthier relationship with food.

5. Nutrient viscosity Choose Wisely

Conclude for nutrient- thick foods that give a high quantum of nutrients relative to their calorie content. Vegetables, fruits, spare proteins, and whole grains are excellent exemplifications.

6. Limit Processed Foods and Added Sugars

Reused foods frequently contain added sugars, unhealthy fats, and redundant sodium. Limiting these particulars reduces empty calorie input and supports overall health.

7. mess Timing thickness Matters

Establishing regular mess times helps regulate hunger and supports metabolism. Aim for balanced refections and snacks throughout the day to maintain energy situations.

8. Be aware of Liquid Calories

Calories from drinks can add up fleetly. Pick water, home grown tea, or other low- calorie choices rather than sweet potables or gratuitous measures of adipose refreshments.

9. Prepare regale Preparation

Arranging feasts ahead of time can avert undiplomatic, undesirable food opinions. Plan nutritional feasts and snacks to have close by, dwindling dependence on comfort food kinds.

10. Pay attention to Your Body Hunger versus jones

Fete genuine hankering and solicitations. Figure out how to perceive when your body really needs food and when outside signals or passions spark a craving to eat.

11. Salutary Fiber Your Stomach related Ally

Integrate fiber-rich food kinds like entire grains, natural products, vegetables, and vegetables into your eating authority. Fiber helps processing, advances a sensation of summation, and supports in general stomach good.

12. Protein's Part in Satiety

Flash back satisfactory protein for your feasts and tidbits. Protein advances a sensation of completion and assists cover with inclining bulk, particularly significant during weight reduction.

13. Balance, Not privation

Take on a intelligence of balance rather of difficulty. Getting a charge out of periodic treats in sensible totalities can help with keeping a practical and acclimated way to deal with eating.   By embracing these aliment rudiments, you establish a strong starting point for a sound way of life and made way for important weight the directors. Keep in mind, it's about what you eat as well as how you approach food that adds to in general substance.

Importance of Portion Control

Member control assumes a vital part in negotiating and keeping a sound weight, advancing generally substance. Then are   crucial reasons featuring the significance of part control

1. Sweet operation

Controlling part measures oversees sweet admission. Consuming a larger number of calories than the body needs can prompt weight gain. By being apprehensive of piece sizes, you make a harmony between energy application and consumption.

2. Weight Management

feasible weight the directors constantly depends on keeping a calorie balance. Member control adds to making a reasonable calorie insufficiency, working with weight reduction or averting overkill weight gain.

3. expectation of Gorging

Bigger parts can prompt indulging, as the mind might get some periphery to matriculate completion. More modest parts consider a superior association between factual malnutrition and food consumption, dwindling the adventure of eating extravagant calories.

4. Glucose Regulation

Conforming member sizes, particularly those containing beans, controls glucose situations. Predictable and controlled corridor can be precious for people overseeing conditions like diabetes or insulin opposition.

5. Stomach related Health

Suitable part measures support solid immersion. Gorging can strain the stomach related frame, egging torture and possible stomach related issues. veritably much controlled parts advance smoother assimilation and supplement ingestion. **

6. Supplement Input

Acclimated parts guarantee an varied admission of supplements from colorful nutritive orders. This is abecedarian for meeting day to day salutary musts, supporting generally speaking good, and averting crunches.

7. Careful Eating

Member control empowers careful eating rehearses. Monitoring how important food you devour encourages a more conscious relationship with food, advancing appreciation for flavors and fulfillment with further modest quantities.

8. Reasonable Habits
Embracing member control as a propensity adds to long haul salutary achievement. It empowers a way of life revolved around balance, making it more probable for people to keep a solid weight and keep down from patterns of prohibitive eating rules followed by intemperance.

9. Mental Impact
More modest parts can in any case be fulfilling when consumed precisely. This acknowledgment can move the intelligence from mate fulfillment simply with enormous quantities to valuing the quality and kinds of food.

10. Social Settings
Controlling bits can be especially profitable in group surroundings where bigger corridor are normal. It permits people to appreciate social events without undermining their good objects.

11. Balance of Plateau
For those on a weight reduction adventure, steady part control forestalls weight reduction situations. As the body changes with a lower sweet admission, observing piece sizes becomes abecedarian for progressed with progress.

12. Long haul Weight conservation

Member control is not only for weight reduction; it's a vital part of keeping a solid cargo over the long run. It lays out provident salutary patterns that can be conveyed forward into day to day actuality. Rehearsing member control is a strong methodology for negotiating and keeping a solid way of life. It upholds weight the directors, controls glucose, upgrades stomach related good, and encourages careful salutary patterns. Integrating member control into your day to day schedule adds to a fair and supportable way to deal with food.

CHAPTER 2
Creating Healthy Habits

Creating healthy habits is integral to long-term well-being and successful weight management. Here's a guide on fostering habits that promote a healthier lifestyle:

1. Start Small:

Begin with manageable changes. Gradual adjustments are more likely to become ingrained habits than attempting a complete overhaul. For example, start by incorporating one additional serving of vegetables into your daily meals.

2. Set Realistic Goals:

Establish achievable goals that align with your lifestyle. Unrealistic expectations can lead to frustration. Break down larger goals into smaller, attainable steps, celebrating each accomplishment along the way.

3. Consistency is Key:

Consistency is the foundation of habit formation. Aim to incorporate healthy behaviors consistently into your daily routine. Whether it's regular exercise, mindful eating, or staying hydrated, repetition reinforces the habit loop.

4. Create a Routine:

Integrate healthy habits into your daily schedule. Establishing a routine makes it easier to incorporate activities like exercise, meal preparation, and adequate sleep into your lifestyle.

5. Identify Triggers:

Recognize the cues or triggers that prompt unhealthy habits. Whether it's stress, boredom, or specific environments, understanding triggers enables you to develop healthier coping mechanisms and responses.

6. Mindful Eating:

Practice mindful eating by being present during meals. Pay attention to hunger and fullness cues, savor each bite, and avoid distractions like screens. This fosters a healthier relationship with food.

7. Plan and Prepare:

Planning meals in advance and having healthy snacks readily available reduces reliance on less nutritious options. Preparation sets the stage for making healthier choices even in busy moments.

8. Incorporate Physical Activity:

Find enjoyable forms of exercise and gradually incorporate them into your routine. Whether it's walking, cycling, or engaging in a fitness class, regular physical activity contributes to overall well-being.

9. Hydration Habits:

Establish a habit of staying hydrated throughout the day. Carry a reusable water bottle, set reminders, or link water consumption to specific daily activities. Hydration supports various bodily functions.

10. Track Progress:
Keep track of your habits and progress. Journaling or using apps can help you monitor your journey, identify patterns, and stay motivated by acknowledging achievements.

11. Seek Social Support:
Engage with friends, family, or communities that share similar health goals. Social support can provide motivation, accountability, and a sense of camaraderie on your journey.

12. Learn from Setbacks:
Recognize that setbacks are a natural part of forming habits. Instead of viewing them as failures, consider them opportunities to learn. Identify the factors that led to the setback and adjust your approach accordingly.

13. Positive Reinforcement:
Celebrate your successes, no matter how small. Positive reinforcement strengthens the neural pathways associated with healthy habits, making them more likely to endure.

14. Prioritize Sleep:

Establish a consistent sleep routine. Quality sleep is foundational to overall health and influences various factors, including hunger hormones and energy levels.

15. Focus on Long-Term Lifestyle:
Shift your mindset from short-term fixes to long-term lifestyle changes. Habits formed with a focus on sustainability are more likely to endure and contribute to lasting well-being.

By incorporating these strategies into your daily life, you can cultivate habits that support a healthier, more balanced lifestyle. Remember, the key lies in consistency, patience, and a positive approach to self-improvement.

Meal Planning and Preparation

Meal planning and preparation are essential factors of a healthy life, abetting in better nutritive choices and time operation. Then is a companion to help you navigate this process effectively

1. Assess Your pretensions and Dietary Needs
Understand your nutritive pretensions, whether it's weight loss, muscle gain, or maintaining overall health. Consider any salutary restrictions or preferences to knitter your mess plan consequently.

2. produce a Weekly or Bi-Weekly Plan

Outline your refections for the forthcoming week or two. This includes breakfast, lunch, regale, and snacks. Planning ahead reduces the liability of impulsive, less healthy food choices.

3. Variety and Balance

Incorporate a variety of foods from different food groups to insure a balanced diet. Include fruits, vegetables, spare proteins, whole grains, and healthy fats in your mess plan.

4. Batch cuisine

Spend some time on batch cuisine during the week or on weekends. Prepare larger amounts of staple particulars like grains, proteins, and vegetables that can be used in multiple refections throughout the week.

5. Choose Simple and Nutrient-thick fashions

conclude for fashions that are easy to prepare and concentrate on nutrient- thick constituents. Look for refections that give a good balance of macronutrients(carbohydrates, proteins, and fats) and micronutrients(vitamins and minerals).

6. Portion Control

Be aware of portion sizes to avoid gluttony. Use measuring tools or visual cues to help gauge applicable serving sizes.

7. Grocery Shopping List

Grounded on your   mess plan,   produce a detailed grocery shopping list. This not only saves time but also helps you stick to your plan when at the store.

8. Stock Up on Healthy Staples

Keep your closet and refrigerator grazed with healthy masses like whole grains, legumes, canned tomatoes, spare proteins, and   firmed   vegetables. This ensures you have the basics for creating nutritional refections.

9. preparing Fresh Produce

Wash, chop, and store fresh fruits and vegetables for easy access. Having them   fixed makes it more likely that you will include them in your refections.

10. Plan for Leftovers

Designedly cook redundant portions to have leavings for unborn   refections. This can save time on days when you may have lower time or energy to cook.

11. Use Time- Saving cuisine styles

Explore cuisine styles that save time, similar as one-visage dishes, slow   cuisine, or   exercising kitchen appliances like a pressure cooker or Instant Pot.

12. Consider Dietary Preferences

Find protean fashions that can be customized, If you are cooking for others with different salutary preferences. For   illustration, have   voluntary condiments or sides for individual preferences.

13. Stay Flexible

While planning is essential, stay flexible. Life happens, and you may need to acclimate your mess plan. Having a plan, still, makes it easier to make healthier choices indeed in unanticipated situations.

14. Plan for Convenience

Include accessible, healthy options for days when you have limited time or energy. This could include pre-packaged salads, whole- grain wraps, or quick- to-assemble refections.

15. Enjoy the Process

View mess planning and medication as a positive and pleasurable part of your routine. trial with new fashions, involve family members, and make it a time to nourish both your body and mind. By incorporating these strategies into your mess planning and medication routine, you can streamline the process and make healthier choices more accessible in your diurnal life.

Mindful Eating Techniques

Careful eating includes being fully present and aware during feasts, cultivating a better relationship with food. Then are styles to rehearse careful eating

1. Slow Down

Eat at a further slow speed, delighting each mouthful. Put your implements down among chomps, and get some periphery to suck and value the flavors and shells of your food.

2. Draw in Your Senses

Pause for a nanosecond to connect with your faculties before you begin eating. Notice the tones, shells, and scents of your food. This makes a more profound association with your regale.

3. Apportion with Distractions

Limit interruptions during feasts. Switch off the TV, set away electronic widgets, and limelight simply on the demonstration of eating. This upgrades knowledge of your body's pining and summation prompts.

4. Pay attention to Your Body

Focus on your body's signs of pining and summation. Eat when you are eager and stop when you are fulfilled. Check out invisible signals as opposed to depending on external rudiments like piece size or external calendars.

5. Registration with feelings

Be apprehensive of close to home eating triggers. Assuming that you end up going after food because of stress, fatigue, or different passions, stop and survey whether eating is the stylish response. suppose about optional strategies for dealing with difficulty or stress.

6. Value Each Bite

Find occasion to see the value in the flavors and shells of each chomp. suck fully and notice the craft in taste. This upgrades the eating experience as well as permits your body to all the more likely commerce the food.

7. Member mindfulness

Be apprehensive of part estimates. use more modest plates, coliseums, and implements to help with controlling corridor. This urges you to eat with end as opposed to carelessly consuming bigger totalities.

8. Eat with Gratitude

Offer thanks for your food. Consider the work that went into delivering and setting up your feast. This positive intelligence can ameliorate your general eating experience.

9. Be Non-Judgmental

Move toward eating without judgment. Try not to name food kinds as" great" or" terrible." All effects considered, center around the salutary benefit and how colorful food sources beget you to feel.

10. Take Breaks

Stop during your feast to survey your degree of completion. This forestalls gorging and permits you to partake in the fulfillment of a veritably important paced regale.

11. Careful Drinking

Stretch out careful eating practices to drinks. Taste your libation gradationally, enjoying each taste. Know about the flavors and how the drink supplements your feast.

12. Careful Snacking

Apply careful eating to snacks. Try not to carelessly crunch before the TV. All effects being equal, member out your bite, flump down, and fully appreciate it.

13. Registration with Hunger

Previous to going after a tidbit or second abetting, check in with your pining situations. Might it be said that you're authentically eager, or is it a response to outside signals? This awareness can avert redundant eating.

14. Consider Food Choices

Consider your food opinions and how they add to your general substance. Consider the salutary benefit of your feasts and how they line up with your good objects.

15. Exercise Gratitude

Offer thanks for the food as well as for the experience of eating. Develop a positive and thankful intelligence towards supporting your body. Integrating these careful eating procedures can change your relationship with food, advancing a more conscious and fascinating way to deal with feasts.

CHAPTER 3
Effective Exercise Routines

Effective exercise routines encompass a combination of cardiovascular, strength training, inflexibility, and balance exercises. Then is a companion to creating a well- rounded and effective drill plan

1. Cardiovascular Exercise   Include conditioning that elevate your heart rate and ameliorate cardiovascular health. Options include ;
Brisk Walking or Jogging
Cycling
Swimming
Jump Rope
Dancing
High- Intensity Interval Training(HIIT)

2. Strength Training
Incorporate exercises that target major muscle groups to make strength and abidance. This can involve ;
Toning
Bodyweight Exercises(e.g., push- ups, syllables, lunges)
Resistance Band exercise
Functional Training(e.g., using stability balls or kettlebells)

3. Inflexibility and Stretching

Ameliorate inflexibility to enhance common range of stir and reduce the   threat of injuries. Include   ;
Stationary Stretching
Dynamic Stretching
Yoga
Pilates

4. Balance Training

Enhance stability and reduce the threat of cascade by incorporating exercises that challenge balance, similar as ;
Single- Leg Stands
Balance Exercises on Unstable shells(e.g., balance pads)
Tai Chi

5. Core Exercises

Strengthening the core is essential for stability and functional movement. Include exercises like ;
Planks
Crunches or Sit- Ups
Russian Twists
Leg Raises

6. Thickness is crucial

Establish a harmonious drill routine. Aim for at least 150 twinkles of moderate- intensity cardio or 75 twinkles of vigorous- intensity cardio per week, along with strength training at least two days per week.

7. Gradational Progression

Progress your exercises gradationally to avoid mesas and reduce the threat of injuries. Increase the intensity, duration, or resistance of your exercises as your fitness position improves.

8. Hear to Your Body

Pay attention to how your body responds to exercise. Allow time for recovery, and if you witness pain or discomfort beyond normal muscle soreness, consult with a healthcare professional.

9. Mix It Up

Avoid humdrum by incorporating variety into your exercises. Try different types of exercises, classes, or out-of-door conditioning to keep effects intriguing and challenge your body in new ways.

10. Warm- Up and Cool Down

Always start your exercises with a proper warm- up to prepare your body for exertion. Include dynamic stretches and movements. Cool down with static stretching to ameliorate inflexibility and reduce muscle pressure.

11. Set Realistic pretensions

Establish attainable fitness pretensions that align with your overall health objects. Whether it's perfecting abidance, structure muscle, or enhancing inflexibility, having clear pretensions provides provocation.

12. Proper Form

Maintain proper form during exercises to maximize effectiveness and help injuries. However, consider working with a fitness professional to insure your form is correct, If doubtful.

13. Include Rest Days
Allow your body time to recover by cataloging regular rest days. Rest is pivotal for muscle form and overall well- being.

14. Stay Doused
Hydration is essential for optimal performance and recovery. Drink water before, during, and after your exercises.

15. hear to Your Preferences
Choose conditioning you enjoy to make exercise a sustainable part of your life. Whether it's hiking, dancing, or toning, chancing conditioning you love increases adherence to your drill routine. Customize your exercise routine grounded on your fitness position, preferences, and any health considerations. thickness and a well- rounded approach are crucial rudiments of an effective and sustainable exercise authority.

Simple Workouts for Beginners
For newcomers, it's important to start with simple and manageable exercises to make a foundation of fitness. Then is a freshman-friendly drill routine that covers

cardiovascular exercise, strength training, inflexibility, and balance

1. Cardiovascular Exercise(20- 30 twinkles)
Brisk Walking
Start with a brisk walk for 20- 30 twinkles. You can do this outside or on a routine. Gradationally increase your pace as you feel more comfortable.

2. Strength Training(2- 3 times per week)
Perform each exercise for 2 sets of 10- 12 reiterations. Start with light weights or resistance and concentrate on proper form.
Bodyweight Squats
Stand with bases shoulder- range piecemeal. -Lower your body by bending your knees and pushing your hips back. - Return to the starting position.
Push- Ups
Begin in a plank position with hands shoulder- range piecemeal. -Lower your body by bending your elbows. - Push back over to the starting position.
Bodyweight Lunges
Step forward with one bottom and lower your body until both knees are fraudulent at a 90- degree angle.
Return to the starting position and switch legs.
Dumbbell Rows(if you have access to dumbbells)
Bend at the hips with a dumbbell in each hand. - Pull the weights toward your casket, squeezing your shoulder blades together.

3. Inflexibility and Stretching(after each drill)
Perform each stretch for 15- 30 seconds, fastening on gentle, controlled movements.
Neck Stretch
Gently cock your head to one side, holding for a many seconds, and also switch.
Shoulder Stretch
Bring one arm across your body, using the contrary hand to gently press on the upper arm.
Hamstring Stretch
Sit or stand with one leg extended and reach toward your toes, keeping your reverse straight.
Casket Nature
Clasp your hands behind your reverse and lift your arms, opening your casket.

4. Balance Exercises(2- 3 times per week)
Single- Leg Stands
Stand on one leg, holding onto a sturdy face if demanded. - Hold for 20- 30 seconds and switch legs.
Heel- to- Toe Walk
Place one bottom in front of the other, touching heel to toe, and walk in a straight line.
Balancing on One Leg with Knee Lift
Lift one knee toward your casket while maintaining balance, also switch legs.

5. Core Exercises(2- 3 times per week)
Perform each exercise for 2 sets of 10- 12 reiterations.
Plank Begin in a forearm plank position, keeping your body in a straight line from head to heels.

Bike Crunches ,taradiddle on your reverse, bring your knees toward your casket, and perform a bicycling stir with your legs while scraping.

Raspberry- Canine - launch on your hands and knees, extend one arm and the contrary leg contemporaneously, also switch sides. Flash back to start at your own pace, gradationally adding intensity and duration as you feel more comfortable. Always consult with a healthcare professional before starting a new exercise routine, especially if you have any health enterprises.

CHAPTER 4
Hydration and its Role

Hydration assumes a vital part in keeping up with generally good and substance. Then are crucial corridor of hydration and its significance

1. Water Balance

Water makes up a critical part of our body, and keeping up with the right equilibrium is abecedarian for different physiological capabilities. It manages internal heat position, upholds processing, and works with supplement transport.

2. Cell Function

Water is a central part of cells, assuming a abecedarian part in cell processes. Applicable hydration guarantees ideal capability of cells, including supplement retention, squander disposal, and synthetic responses.

3. Temperature Regulation

Perspiring is the body's normal element for chilling off. Remaining doused directs internal heat position by supporting the perspiring system during factual work or in hot conditions.

4. Mental Function

Parchedness can negatively affect internal capability. Indeed, indeed gentle lack of hydration might prompt challenges in focus, readiness, and flash memory.

Remaining sufficiently doused is critical for ideal mind capability.

5. Factual Performance

Applicable hydration is essential for athletic prosecution. Lack of hydration can prompt prostration, muscle squeezes, and impaired perseverance. Challengers should keep up with ideal liquid situations to help maximum prosecution.

6. Common Lubrication

Water is a part of synovial liquid, which greases up joints. Remaining doused keeps up with common good and can reduce torture related with parchedness.

7. Supplement Transport

Water goes about as a transporter for supplements, moving them all through the body. This is abecedarian for the assimilation and dispersion of supplements from the stomach related frame to cells.

8. Detoxification

Hydration is vital for the feathers and liver, which assume a crucial part in detoxifying the body. Acceptable water consumption upholds the end of derivations and venoms through pee.

9. Skin Health

Applicable hydration adds to skin good and appearance. Got dried out skin might come dry, short, and more inclined to early growing. Drinking sufficient water keeps up with skin versatility and a solid tone.

10. Electrolyte Balance

Electrolytes, like sodium, potassium, and magnesium, assume a abecedarian part in liquid equilibrium and cell capability. Hydration keeps up with the licit equilibrium of electrolytes in the body.

11. Stomach related Health

Sufficient water admission is abecedarian for processing. It helps separate food, assimilate supplements, and move squander through the intestinal system. shy hydration can prompt cessation and other stomach related issues.

12. State of mind and Energy

Lack of hydration can add to sensations of weariness and low energy situations. Remaining doused upholds by and large essentialness and can substantially affect disposition and energy situations.

13. Weight Management

Drinking water before feasts can add to a sensation of completion, conceivably supporting weight the board by dwindling generally calorie consumption.

14. Averting Dehumidification

It's essential to proactively keep up with hydration rather of holding on until you feel parched. Thirst is an suggestion that your body is now kindly dried out.

15. Individual requirements

Hydration needs shift among people and can be impacted by variables, for illustration, age, movement position, terrain, and in general good. Focus on your body's signs and change your water consumption as requirements be. Applicable hydration is abecedarian for ideal physical processes, from supporting cell cycles to keeping up with internal capability and generally speaking substance. Growing great hydration propensities is an essential part of a solid way of life.

Tips for Increasing Water Intake

Adding water input is a simple yet poignant way to enhance overall health. Then are tips to help you drink further water throughout the day

1. Carry a Water Bottle

Keep a applicable water bottle with you wherever you go. Having water readily available makes it more likely that you will take regular drafts.

2. Set monuments

Use your phone or other electronic bias to set monuments at intervals throughout the day to drink water. This can help establish a routine.

3. Flavor Your Water

If plain water does not excite you, try investing it with slices of fruits, similar as bomb, cucumber, or berries. This adds flavor without added sugars or calories.

4. Establish Drinking Habits

Make it a habit to drink water at certain times, similar as when you wake up, before refections, and before bedtime. Creating routines can make hydration more harmonious.

5. Use an App

Consider using a hydration app that tracks your water input and sends monuments. Some apps also give individualized recommendations grounded on factors like age, weight, and exertion position.

6. Drink Before refections

Have a glass of water before each mess. Not only does this contribute to your diurnal input, but it can also help control appetite and help gluttony.

7. Track Your Input

Keep track of your diurnal water consumption in a journal or a moblle app. This can help you cover your progress and identify patterns in your hydration habits.

8. Make It a Challenge

Challenge yourself to drink a certain quantum of water each day. You can set diurnal or daily pretensions and award yourself when you achieve them.

9. Eat Hydrating Foods

Consume foods with high water content, similar as watermelon, cucumber, celery, and oranges. These foods contribute to your overall hydration. **

10. Replace Other potables

Gradually replace sticky drinks and caffeinated potables with water. This not only increases your water input but also reduces your consumption of lower healthy options.

11. Adulterate sticky Drinks

If you enjoy sticky drinks, adulterate them with water to reduce the sugar content while still enjoying the flavor.

12. Examiner Urine Color

Pay attention to the color of your urine. Light unheroic or pale straw color generally indicates acceptable hydration, while dark yellow may suggest dehumidification.

13. Use a Straw

Drinking through a straw can make it more pleasurable and may encourage you to drink further water throughout the day.

14. produce a Hydration Station

Keep water fluently accessible in places where you spend the utmost time, whether it's your office, kitchen, or living room.

15. Set pretensions for Increased Input

Gradationally increase your diurnal water input by setting realistic goals .However, aim to add an redundant glass each day until you reach your target, If you are presently drinking lower water. Flash back that individual hydration requirements vary, so it's essential to hear to your body and acclimate your water input grounded on factors like exertion position, climate, and overall health. Developing harmonious habits will contribute to a more doused and healthier you.

CHAPTER 5
Sleep and Stress Management

Sleep and stress   operation are integral   factors of overall well- being. Then are tips for   perfecting both areas   Sleep Management

1. harmonious Sleep Schedule
Go to bed and wake up at the same time every day, indeed on weekends. thickness reinforces your body's natural sleep- wake cycle.

2. Produce a Relaxing Bedtime Routine
Develop a pre-sleep routine to gesture to your body that it's time to wind down. This could include conditioning like reading, gentle stretching, or harkening to calming music.

3. Comfortable Sleep Environment
Insure your bedroom is conducive to sleep. Keep it dark, quiet, and cool. Invest in a comfortable mattress and pillows.

4. Limit Exposure to Screens Before Bed
Avoid electronic bias with defenses at least an hour before bedtime. The blue light emitted can intrude with the product of the sleep hormone melatonin.

5. Watch Your Diet

Avoid heavy refections, caffeine, and nicotine close to bedtime. conclude for a light snack if you are empty before bed.

6. Regular Exercise
Engage in regular physical exertion, but avoid vigorous exercise close to bedtime. Exercise promotes better sleep, but timing matters.

7. Manage Stress
Practice stress- reducing ways, similar as contemplation, deep breathing, or progressive muscle relaxation, to calm your mind before bedtime.

8. Limit Naps
If you need to nap, keep it short(20- 30 twinkles) and before in the day to avoid snooping with darkness sleep.

9. Estimate Your Mattress and Pillows
Insure that your mattress and pillows give proper support. An uncomfortable sleep terrain can contribute to poor sleep quality.

10. Get Exposure to Natural Light
Spend time outside during daylight hours. Natural light exposure helps regulate your body's internal timepiece.

Stress operation ;
1. Identify Stressors

Fete and identify sources of stress in your life. Understanding what triggers stress is the first step in managing it effectively.

2. Prioritize and Organize

Break down tasks into manageable way. Prioritize what needs to be done and concentrate on one thing at a time to avoid feeling overwhelmed.

3. Time Management

Plan your day efficiently. Set realistic pretensions, and allocate time for breaks and relaxation. Avoid overcommitting yourself. **

4. Learn to Say No

Understand your limits and be willing to say no when you need to. Overcommitting can lead to increased stress. **

5. Exercise awareness

Engage in awareness practices, similar as contemplation or yoga, to bring your attention to the present moment and reduce anxiety about the future.

6. Stay Connected

Maintain social connections with musketeers and family. Having a support system can give emotional support during stressful times.

7. Physical exertion

Regular exercise is a important stress reliever. Find conditioning you enjoy, whether it's walking, jogging, dancing, or yoga.

8. Healthy life Choices

Prioritize a healthy life with a balanced diet, regular exercise, and acceptable sleep. A well- nourished body is better equipped to handle stress.

9. Seek Professional Help

If stress becomes inviting, consider seeking support from an internal health professional. remedy can give precious tools for managing stress.

10. Exercise Relaxation ways

Incorporate relaxation ways into your diurnal routine, similar as deep breathing, progressive muscle relaxation, or guided imagery. Balancing sleep and stress operation contributes significantly to overall physical and internal well- being. enforcing these strategies can help produce a foundation for a healthier and further flexible life.

CHAPTER 6
Smart Snacking

Smart snacking involves making nutritional and satisfying choices that give energy and support overall well- being. Then are tips for smart snacking

1. Choose Nutrient-thick Foods

Opt for snacks that are rich in nutrients, similar as fruits, vegetables, whole grains, nuts, seeds, and dairy products. These foods give essential vitamins, minerals, and fiber.

2. Combine Macronutrients

Produce balanced snacks by combining macronutrients protein, carbohydrates, and healthy fats. This combination helps keep you fuller for longer and provides sustained energy.

3. Portion Control

Be aware of portion sizes. Indeed healthy snacks can contribute to redundant calorie input if consumed in large amounts. Use small coliseums or holders to control portions.

4. Include Protein

Protein-rich snacks help promote malnutrition and muscle form. Good protein sources include Greek yogurt, nut adulation, hummus, and spare flesh.

5. Fiber- Rich Choices

Fiber aids in digestion and helps you feel satisfied. Choose snacks with high fiber content, similar as whole fruits, vegetables, nuts, and whole grains.

6. Hydrate

Stay doused by pairing your snacks with water or herbal tea. Thirst is occasionally incorrect for hunger, so staying doused can help gratuitous snacking.

7. Plan Ahead

Prepare healthy snacks in advance. Having nutritional options readily available reduces the temptation to reach for less healthy druthers

8. Snack Mindfully

Pay attention to hunger cues and eat when you are authentically empty. Avoid gorging out of tedium or stress. Exercise aware eating by savoring each bite. **

9. Choose Whole Foods

Opt for whole, minimally reused foods over largely reused snacks. Whole foods give further nutritive value and smaller added sugars and preservatives. **

10. Healthy Sweet Treats

If you have a sweet tooth, choose healthier sweet options like fresh fruit, yogurt with honey, or a small piece of dark chocolate.

11. Trail Mix with Variety

Produce your own trail blend with a blend of nuts, seeds, dried fruits, and a hint of dark chocolate. This combination offers a balance of nutrients and flavors.

12. Vegetable Sticks with Hummus

Enjoy sliced vegetables like cucumber, carrot, and bell pepper with a side of hummus. This provides a satisfying crunch along with fiber and protein.

13. Greek Yogurt Parfait

Subcaste Greek yogurt with fresh berries and a sprinkle of granola. It's a succulent and nutritional snack that combines protein, vitamins, and whole grains.

14. Rubbish and Whole Grain Crackers

Brace a small portion of rubbish with whole grain crackers for a satisfying snack that combines protein and complex carbohydrates.

15. Air- Popped Popcorn

Choose air- popped popcorn as a whole- grain, fiber-rich snack. You can customize it with a sprinkle of sauces or nutritive incentive for flavor.   Smart snacking involves making purposeful choices that align with your nutritive pretensions. By opting nutrient- thick foods, rehearsing portion control, and paying attention to your body's hunger cues, you can enjoy snacks that contribute to your overall health and well- being.

Healthy Snack Options

Then are some healthy snack options that are nutritional, satisfying, and easy to incorporate into your diurnal routine

1. Fresh Fruit

Apples, bananas, berries, oranges, or any seasonal fruit are excellent choices. They give vitamins, minerals, and natural sugars for a quick energy boost.

2. Greek Yogurt

Greek yogurt is rich in protein and probiotics. Choose straight,nonfat or low-fat options, and add fresh fruit, nuts, or a mizzle of honey for flavor.

3. Nuts and Seeds

Almonds, walnuts, chia seeds, or pumpkin seeds are nutrient- thick snacks rich in healthy fats, protein, and fiber. Enjoy them in temperance due to their calorie viscosity.

4. Vegetable Sticks with Hummus

Carrot, cucumber, bell pepper, or celery sticks paired with hummus make a brickle and a satisfying snack. Hummus provides protein and healthy fats.

5. Nut Adulation and Whole Grain Crackers

Spread almond adulation, peanut adulation, or cashew adulation on whole grain crackers for a combination of protein, healthy fats, and complex carbohydrates.

6. Hard- Boiled Eggs

Hard- boiled eggs are a accessible and protein- packed snack. Sprinkle them with a pinch of swab and pepper for flavor.

7. Cabin rubbish with Pineapple

Cabin rubbish paired with fresh pineapple gobbets creates a delicious and protein-rich snack. It's a good blend of protein and natural agreeableness.

8. Avocado Toast

Top whole grain toast with mashed avocado and a sprinkle of swab and pepper. This snack provides healthy fats and fiber.

9. Air- Popped Popcorn

Popcorn is a whole- grain snack when prepared without inordinate adulation or oil painting. Air- pop your popcorn and season it with sauces or nutritive incentive for flavor.

10. Dark Chocolate and Almonds

A small portion of dark chocolate(70 cocoa or advanced) paired with almonds offers a satisfying blend of antioxidants, healthy fats, and protein.

11. Fresh Berries with cabin rubbish

Combine fresh berries with cabin rubbish for a succulent and nutrient-rich snack that provides a balance of protein and antioxidants.

12. Rice galettes with Nut Adulation

Spread nut adulation on whole grain rice galettes for a satisfying and movable snack. It's a good combination of protein and complex carbohydrates.

13. Edamame
Steamed edamame(youthful soybeans) is a protein-rich snack that also provides fiber. Sprinkle with a pinch of ocean swab for added flavor.

14. Veggie Slices with Guacamole
Dip cucumber, bell pepper, or cherry tomatoes in guacamole for a delicious snack rich in healthy fats, vitamins, and minerals.

15. Green Smoothie
Mix spinach or kale with a banana, Greek yogurt, and a splash of almond milk for a nutrient- packed green smoothie.   Flash back to knitter your snacks to your preferences and salutary requirements. These options give a balance of macronutrients and micronutrients to keep you fueled and satisfied between refections.

Avoiding Mindless Eating

Avoiding Careless eating involves cultivating awareness and making purposeful choices about what and when you eat. Then are strategies to help you break the habit of careless eating

1. Eat Without Distractions

Avoid eating in front of the television, computer, or while scrolling through your phone. Focus on the sensitive experience of eating to enhance satisfaction and mindfulness.

2. Use lower Plates and coliseums

Opt for lower dishware to control portion sizes. Research suggests that people tend to eat further when using larger plates, as it may produce a perception of a lower portion.

3. Portion Control

Be aware of serving sizes. Use measuring tools or visual cues to avoid over-serving yourself, especially with snacks.

4. Hear to Hunger Cues

Pay attention to your body's hunger and wholeness signals. Eat when you are empty, and stop when you are satisfied. Avoid eating out of tedium or for emotional reasons.

5. Exercise aware Eating

Engage in aware eating by savoring each bite. Notice the flavors, textures, and sensations of the food. Put your chopstick down between mouthfuls to decelerate down the eating process.

6. Plan refections and Snacks

Plan your refections and snacks in advance. Having a structured eating schedule can reduce impulsive and careless eating.

7. Keep Unhealthy Snacks Out of Sight
Store unhealthy snacks in less accessible places and keep healthier options visible. This simple change can impact snack choices.

8. Slow Down
Bite your food sluggishly and enjoy each bite. Eating too snappily may lead to gluttony, as your body may not have enough time to gesture wholeness.

9. Be aware of Emotional Eating
Be   apprehensive of emotional triggers that lead to eating. Find indispensable ways to manage with stress, tedium, or other feelings, similar as going for a walk or rehearsing deep breathing.

10. Hydrate Before refections
Drink water before refections. Thirst is occasionally incorrect for hunger, and staying doused can help control appetite.

11. Keep a Food Journal
Track your refections and snacks in a food journal. This can increase mindfulness of eating patterns and help identify careless eating triggers.

12. Enjoy Balanced refections

Produce balanced refections that include a blend of protein, healthy fats, and carbohydrates. This balance can help keep you satisfied and help gluttony latterly.

13. Avoid Eating Straight from the Package
Portion out snacks onto a plate or coliseum rather of eating directly from the package. This makes it easier to control portions.

14. Know Your Alarms
Identify situations or surroundings that spark careless eating. Develop strategies to navigate these situations without counting on food.

15. Be Kind to Yourself
Practice   tone-compassion.However, admit it without judgment and direct on making aware choices moving forward, If you find yourself engaging in careless eating. By incorporating these strategies into your diurnal routine, you can develop a further aware approach to eating. Cultivating   mindfulness around your eating habits and making purposeful choices contributes to a healthier relationship with food.

CHAPTER 7
Tracking Progress

Following headway is fundamental for remaining inspired and settling on informed choices on your excursion, whether it's connected with wellness, wellbeing, or individual objectives. Here are successful ways of keeping tabs on your development:

1. Set Clear Goals:

Characterize explicit, quantifiable, reachable, pertinent, and time-bound (Shrewd) objectives. Having clear targets gives you a system for following advancement.

2. Keep a Journal:

Keep a diary to record your day to day exercises, sentiments, and accomplishments. This can give bits of knowledge into examples and assist you with remaining responsible.

3. Take Standard Measurements:

Track actual changes by estimating key measurements like weight, body estimations, or muscle versus fat ratio. Utilize a predictable technique and timetable for precise examinations.

4. Use Wellness Apps:

Influence wellness applications and trackers to screen exercises, nourishment, and generally action. Numerous applications give diagrams and charts to imagine progress over the long run.

5. Take Progress Photos:

Catch photographs at customary spans to archive changes in your constitution outwardly. This can be a strong method for seeing change that probably won't be obvious in numbers alone.

6. Record Individual Records:

Monitor individual records in your exercises. Whether it's lifting heavier loads, running longer distances, or accomplishing quicker times, taking note of enhancements helps inspiration.

7. Screen Wellbeing Metrics:

Track wellbeing pointers, for example, circulatory strain, cholesterol levels, and resting pulse. Talk with medical services experts for standard check-ups.

8. Think about Achievements:

Celebrate accomplishments, regardless of how little. Considering progress supports positive ways of behaving and inspires you to proceed.

9. Lay out a Standard Check-In:

Set customary stretches for progress appraisals. This could be week by week, fortnightly, or month to month, contingent upon your objectives. Steady registrations give important information.

10. Make a Visual Advancement Board:
Plan a visual board or diagram showing your objectives and progress. Place it in a noticeable area as an everyday update and wellspring of inspiration.

11. Share Your Goals:
Discuss your objectives with a companion, relative, or a strong local area. Sharing your process can give consolation and responsibility.

12. Change Objectives as Needed:
Be adaptable with your objectives. Assuming conditions change or you experience startling difficulties, change your goals while remaining fixed on progress.

13. Assess and Learn:
Consistently assess what's working and what needs change. Gain from the two triumphs and mishaps to refine your methodology.

14. Keep an Appreciation Journal:
Incorporate an appreciation practice into your following. Recognizing positive parts of your process improves inspiration and in general prosperity.

15. Embrace Non-Scale Victories:
Perceive and celebrate non-scale triumphs, for example, further developed energy levels, better rest, or expanded certainty. These markers are similarly pretty much as significant as mathematical information.

Predictable following gives significant criticism and assists you with remaining on track. Recollect that progress is frequently nonlinear, and the excursion might include high points and low points. Show restraint, remain on track, and praise the little wins en route.

Keeping a Food Journal

Keeping a food journal is an amazing asset for acquiring understanding into your salutary patterns, advancing care, and negotiating healthy objects. This is the reason and the way to successfully keep a food journal

Why Keep a Food Journal

1. Mindfulness
A food journal carries attention to what, when, and why you eat. It recognizes exemplifications and triggers, encouraging a more profound appreciation of your relationship with food.

2. Member Control
Recording member sizes assists you with turning out to be more apprehensive of serving sizes and forestalls indulging.

3. Supplement Input
Following feasts permits you to screen your supplement admission. You can guarantee you are getting a decent

eating routine with the abecedarian nutrients, minerals, and macronutrients.

4. Responsibility
A food journal considers you responsible for your opinions. It tends to be a wellspring of alleviation to settle on better choices.

5. Fete Profound Eating
Perceive close to home triggers for eating. Following your mind- set and conditions around feasts can uncover assuming you are eating because of passions as opposed to hunger.

6. Track Progress
On the off chance that you have unequivocal good or heartiness objects, a food journal helps keep tabs on your development and change your eating routine as requirements be. **

7. Lay out Solid Habits
It supports shaping and erecting up smart overeating propensities. Steady following adds to the advancement of careful and purposeful eating. **

Instructions to Keep a Food Journal
1. Pick a Format
Conclude whether you favor an factual journal, a protean operation, or a motorized computation distance. Pick a configuration that suits your way of life and inclinations.

2. Record instantly

Record your feasts and snacks at the foremost occasion in the wake of eating. This guarantees fineness and forestalls neglecting craft.

3. Incorporate Details

For every passage, incorporate   craft, for   illustration, the kind of food, member size, cooking ways, and any seasoning or setoffs.

4. Note regale Times

Record the time you eat every feast. This can help with identifying designs in your eating plan.

5. Track potables

Incorporate refreshments like water, tea, espresso, and any amalgamations. Hydration is a abecedarian part of generally good.   **

6. Record Close to home Factors

Note your close to home state and any outside factors affecting your eating   opinions. This can uncover associations among disposition and salutary patterns.

7. Be Honest

Be straightforward with yourself and record all that you eat. The design is tone- reflection, not judgment.

8. Use Part Sizes

Figure out how to   estimate member measures precisely. Over the long run, you will turn out to be more artful at checking serving sizes without taking estimating instruments.

9. Survey Regularly

Put away occasion to routinely review your food journal. Search for patterns, distinguish regions for development, and celebrate palms.

10. Look for Guidance

In the event that you have unequivocal good or salutary objects, consider talking with an enrolled dietitian or nutritionist. They can give direction in light of your food journal passages.

11. Redo for Your pretensions

Conform your food journal to line up with your objects. For weight the directors, center around calories and macronutrients. On the off chance that you are holding back nothing, emphasize colorful supplement rich food sources.

12. Test and Acclimate

Use the food journal to try different effects with colorful eating exemplifications or salutary changes. See what these changes mean for your substance and change depending on the situation. Keeping a food journal is an individual excursion. It's tied in with acquiring gests into your remarkable relationship with food and exercising that information to make educated, positive opinions.

CHAPTER 8
Looking Ahead to a Healthier Futures

As we journey into the future, embracing a healthier lifestyle becomes not only a goal but a commitment to overall well-being. Here are key aspects to focus on as you look ahead to a healthier future:

1. Mindful Nutrition:
Cultivate a mindful approach to eating. Focus on nourishing your body with nutrient-dense foods, savoring each bite, and paying attention to hunger and fullness cues.

2. Regular Physical Activity:
Integrate regular exercise into your routine. Find activities you enjoy, whether it's walking, cycling, dancing, or yoga. Physical activity not only benefits your body but also enhances mental well-being.

3. Holistic Well-being:
   - Prioritize holistic well-being by addressing mental, emotional, and physical health. Incorporate stress-reducing practices like meditation, deep breathing, and adequate sleep.

4. Personalized Wellness Goals:

Set personalized wellness goals that align with your values and aspirations. Whether it's weight management, improved fitness, or enhanced mental health, tailor your goals to reflect your unique journey.

5. Hydration Habits:
- Maintain optimal hydration by consistently drinking water throughout the day. Hydration plays a crucial role in supporting various bodily functions.

6. Balanced Meal Planning:
Embrace balanced meal planning. Strive for a variety of colorful fruits, vegetables, lean proteins, whole grains, and healthy fats. Experiment with flavors and cooking methods to keep meals enjoyable.

7. Lifelong Learning:
Foster a mindset of lifelong learning about nutrition, fitness, and overall well-being. Stay informed about the latest research and wellness practices to make informed choices.

8. Building Resilience:
Cultivate resilience in the face of challenges. Understand that setbacks are a natural part of any journey, and use them as opportunities to learn and grow.

9. Connection and Community:
Nurture connections with others and build a supportive community. Whether through friends, family, or online

networks, a sense of community can provide encouragement and motivation.

10. Restorative Sleep:
Prioritize quality sleep. Create a sleep-friendly environment, establish a consistent bedtime routine, and ensure you get the recommended hours of rest each night.

11. Joyful Movement:
Approach physical activity as joyful movement. Find activities that bring joy and satisfaction, making exercise an integral part of your lifestyle rather than a chore.

12. Mind-Body Practices:
Explore mind-body practices such as yoga or tai chi. These practices not only contribute to physical health but also promote mental clarity and emotional well-being.

13. Gratitude and Positivity:
- Cultivate a mindset of gratitude and positivity. Recognize and appreciate the positive aspects of your health journey, fostering a sense of optimism for the future.

14. Regular Health Check-ups:
Schedule regular health check-ups and screenings. Proactive healthcare contributes to early detection and prevention of potential health issues.

15. Environmental Awareness:

Be mindful of your impact on the environment. Make sustainable choices in your diet and lifestyle that not only benefit your health but also contribute to a healthier planet.

Looking ahead to a healthier future involves continuous commitment, self-compassion, and a willingness to adapt. Embrace the journey, celebrate achievements, and keep striving for a life filled with vitality and well-being.

Conclusion

Charting Your Course to a Healthier You with the Weight Loss Beginners Diet 2024

As we draw the curtain on our exploration of the Weight Loss Beginners Diet 2024, it's evident that this journey is not just about shedding pounds; it's a transformative path towards a healthier and more vibrant version of yourself.

Reflecting on Key Insights:

1. Sustainable Change: The Weight Loss Beginners Diet 2024 isn't a quick fix; it's a blueprint for sustainable change. It guides you towards establishing habits that will endure, fostering lasting well-being.

2. Mindful Choices: Central to this approach is the concept of mindful choices. Whether it's savoring nutrient-rich meals, engaging in enjoyable physical activities, or being conscious of emotional triggers, mindfulness becomes your compass.

3. Personal Empowerment: The diet empowers you to make personalized decisions. It recognizes that every individual is unique, and encourages you to tailor the plan to your preferences, ensuring that your journey aligns with your lifestyle.

4. Gradual Progress: This isn't a race; it's a gradual progression towards a healthier you. Small, consistent steps, be it in meal planning, physical activity, or self-care, accumulate to create a significant impact over time.

As you look ahead on this journey, remember that success isn't solely measured by the numbers on a scale. It's found in the newfound energy, the enhanced mood, and the overall sense of well-being that accompanies a healthier lifestyle.

Celebrate the victories, both big and small, and learn from any challenges. Your commitment to this path is a testament to your dedication to a healthier and more fulfilling future.

So, here's to the next chapter—filled with mindful meals, invigorating activities, and the ongoing discovery of a healthier, happier you. The Weight Loss Beginners Diet 2024 is not just a plan; it's a guide for the transformative journey you've embarked upon. May it lead you to a future where health is not a destination but a way of life.

About the Author

Dr. Sharon S. Lent

Welcome to the realm of sustainable weight loss and nourishing diets! **Dr. Lent**, a seasoned medical professional specializing in weight loss and diet, brings a wealth of expertise to guide you on your transformative journey to a healthier you.

Meet Dr. Sharon S. Lent

With a passion for empowering individuals to achieve their health goals, **Dr. Sharon S. Lent** has dedicated her career to the intersection of medicine, nutrition, and well-being. Holding a Doctor of Medicine degree, her specialized focus on weight loss has allowed her to make a meaningful impact on countless lives.

Areas of Expertise

Dr. Lent is renowned for her comprehensive approach to weight management, combining medical knowledge with practical, sustainable strategies. Her expertise includes personalized diet plans, evidence-based interventions, and holistic well-being practices.

A Trusted Guide:

As a trusted guide on the journey to better health, **Dr. Lent** emphasizes the importance of mindful living, making choices that resonate with individual lifestyles, and fostering a positive relationship with food.

Contributions to the Field:

Beyond her clinical practice, **Dr. Lent** is an avid contributor to the field of weight management. Her research, articles, and contributions to reputable health publications reflect a commitment to sharing knowledge and fostering a community dedicated to wellness.

Join the Journey:

Embark on a journey towards sustainable weight loss and a nourished, balanced life with **Dr. Lent**. Through her insights, you'll discover practical, achievable steps that go beyond the conventional approach to dieting, paving the way for a healthier, more vibrant future.

Review

Dear **Reader**,

We hope you're enjoying your journey with the Weight Loss Beginners Diet 2024! Your experience matters to us, and we'd love to hear your thoughts on how the program has been for you.

Whether you've just started or are well into your transformation, your review can inspire others and help us fine-tune our approach to better suit your needs. Please take a moment to share your feedback on the Weight Loss Beginners Diet 2024. Your insights are invaluable in shaping the success stories of our community.

Thank you for being a part of this journey with us. Your review is not just a reflection of your experience but also a beacon for others seeking a healthier lifestyle.

We appreciate your time and input.

www.ingramcontent.com/pod-product-compliance
Lightning Source LLC
Chambersburg PA
CBHW071055260726

48661CB00006B/2283